16 U

How the discovery of diabetes changed my life in 10 days

This is intended to be a self-help book as well as a of the unknown world of diabetes.

This book tells the true story of the story's protagonist, whose real name has been changed for privacy reasons.

In it, the author recounts everything the story's protagonist experienced in just 10 days. Ten days that turned into a real hell, ten days that almost led to the protagonist's death.

Ten days of discovery, ten days of fright, ten days of turning points, ten days of preparing for a new life, a new start.

To Prof. Doctor Guilhermina Rego, my Heartfelt thanks to a friend, a sensational person, who helped me through this terrible time and whose words encouragement and strength gave me made us believe and overcome this moment.

Thanks also to Professor Tiago Sousa Veloso, the ACP doctor who saved my life.

The Author

Chapter 1

Carlota Cardoso was a cheerful, good-natured person, always ready to help people, very loyal and faithful to her friends, and if necessary she would take off her shirt to give to others.

She was 58 years old, a law degree and a master's degree in commercial law and was also a specialist in tax law.
Practiced law for many years, worked for ten years in Madrid for one of the largest law firms in the Iberian Peninsula and was currently a legal consultant for some lawyers and also for several companies in the Vale do Ave area and the Tãmega e Sousa area, mainly footwear, footwear components and home textiles companies.

She led a very busy life, full of work, as well as having another activity that she loved, which was writing.

He had already published several books, in a variety of different genres, from romances to thrillers. But what really gave him the most pleasure was writing novels, love stories, some with happy endings, others not, but realistic and mainly where women played the leading role. Carlota was a romantic and always would be, but never a love-story.

She always wrote about powerful women, often women who suffered but always came out victorious and heroines.

Of course, all this activity caused him a lot of stress, a lot of anxiety, as he always had many deadlines to meet and even in his writing.

Then there were the many problems that the companies I worked for had to face, which were sometimes difficult to solve, but I always managed to do it, with hard work, dedication and effort.

I always had a lot of contracts to draw up, agency contracts, representation contracts, always written in Portuguese and English, always having to speak at least three foreign languages, Spanish, English and French. I also had a lot of questions and

tax law cases relating to those same companies. And there were very few lawyers and jurists specializing in this branch of law in Portugal.

I also did a lot of international law, and often had to go to Strasbourg or The Hague, where the European Court of Human Rights and the International Court of Justice were located.

This was Carlota's life, filled with her dogs, her mother and her sister Helena, the person she loved most in the world.

Carlota was single, a choice she made after her long-term boyfriend died of a long-term illness, 28 years ago.

But Carlota closed herself off from the world and closed herself off from love. She thought Fernando was irreplaceable, there would never be anyone like him, and the comparisons with other men she met were the main reason she wanted to remain single.

Comparisons were poison, they were Carlota's perfect enemy. That's why she thought she was doing well and wanted to carry on.

Chapter 2

June 2024

Carlota was very anxious about a complicated deadline and had also just had a setback with a lawyer who worked for her and who suddenly decided to leave complaining that she was having a lot of financial difficulties and earning well, she thought she was earning too little and always wanted more.

Carlota paid him well, but it still wasn't enough. He filled his helmet and they decided to dissolve the partnership.

And Carlota's luck was that with the summer judicial vacation approaching, she would have time to find a replacement, but she still suffered complete ingratitude from the other lawyer, after everything she had done for her.

He later came to the sad conclusion that she didn't like working and wanted easy money.

What is certain is that he left Carlota in the lurch, with even more worries and problems.

In fact, it wasn't until half a dozen weeks later that Carlota realized how much this situation had affected her mentally, psychologically and even physically.

Carlota began to lose a lot of weight, eat little and feel very tired. But she completely dismissed these symptoms. She attributed them to the stress she had been experiencing.

And so his life continued, and in July 2024 he decided to work with other lawyers, with whom he had worked before and whom he had known for more than twenty years, and who thus replaced the previous one, and for the better.

After the judicial vacation, Carlota continued to work at 100% and in midOctober she began to experience daily heartburn that made her feel very ill. She asked her sister to put her on a diet, thinking it would go away, but it didn't.

But I didn't want to see a doctor. I was afraid, very afraid.

A few more days passed and Carlota, already exhausted, turned to her sister Helena and said: - One day Helena is going to give me a stroke or something, you'll see.

Helena, already furious with the situation, simply replied: "Go to the doctor, won't you, what do you want to do?

November 2024

November 3rd, 2024

Carlota and her sister spent the day in Vila Real, at the home of a friend and client of Carlota's.

The three adored each other. It was a healthy and beautiful friendship.

Lunchtime came and, as they always did, they chose a good restaurant to eat in.

This time the chosen restaurant was "Cais da Vila", which had a Michelin recommendation.

Carlota had been there before and really enjoyed it. The food was tasty and well prepared and the desserts and wines were fantastic.

Carlota was a connoisseur of good wines, she really knew a lot, and she had a client who was a famous wine maker, Douro wines, among other well-known people who also made excellent wines.

And she even began to like Douro wines more, which until then had been neglected by Carlota for the famous Alentejo wines.

They had fabulous starters, then monkfish rice as their main course, and then a divine dessert of sponge cake, soft eggs, ice cream and "syrup" with forest fruits.

-Wow! said Carlota.

Dessert was a real calorie bomb. Carlota knew this but what the hell, she was a glutton, she loved sweets, ice cream and chocolates.

Not her sister, she was completely averse to sweets. She was always warning Carlota to be careful, but she didn't care.

One day, some misfortune would happen and Carlota couldn't imagine how much it would affect her life.

Chapter 3

The terrible ten days

November 4th, 2024

It was a Monday and Carlota's sister had gone to do some work her daughter's house, who lived near them and had a small shoe sewing factory.

Carlota stayed at home alone, but she felt increasingly unwell. To make matters worse, she had scrambled eggs and soup for lunch and drank water from rocks.

Scrambled eggs, Carlota? After yesterday?" Carlota's conscience snarled to itself.

At around sixteen o'clock, Carlota was struck by a terrible frontal headache, right in the middle of her forehead, but so horrible that she started screaming and putting her hands on her head.

-Hey Helena, I can't stand it, I feel like my head is going to be ripped off. I feel like I'm having a stroke.

And suddenly he started vomiting non-stop.

There was no end to vomiting, it seemed like a river was coming out of Carlota's mouth.

More and more water was coming out, yellow water. God, what was that?" thought Carlota.

He went to bed but it was use. She threw up every few minutes, constantly. Carlota didn't know where she had so much water inside her to vomit like that.

That same night he vomited non-stop. His stomach, belly and head hurt more and more.

November 5th, 2024

Tuesday was a day to forget and much worse than the previous one.

Carlota hardly ate anything, what she did eat she threw up, even white diet soup. She vomited constantly until, at around 5pm, she turned to her sister and finally said, after trying so hard to resist: -

Helena, please take me to a hospital, I can't stand it any longer. Tears streamed down Carlota's face, thick tears falling one by one like raindrops.

Helena immediately called a cab, and fifteen minutes later they were at the Agostinho Ribeiro Hospital in Felgueiras, in the emergency room. Carlota was

She had a cane, but still couldn't hold on, so they went to get her a wheelchair.

Four hours passed and at 10 p.m. Carlota was seen by a doctor, who was unfortunately not very attentive.

Diagnosis: - You have gastroenteritis. Go and take a bottle of saline and you'll be fine.

Carlota stayed in a chair, taking an IV for another two hours. When the serum was finished, she waited another half an hour, then went back to the same doctor, who prescribed some medicine for her nausea and off she went.

He returned home by cab at 2am.

Carlota kept a sort of professional and personal diary in her diary. She wrote down everything that happened each day, from the moment she got up until the moment she went to bed. She always, always did. And as a woman of faith, she always ended by thanking Jesus for the day, good or bad.

At that time, two in the morning, she got home, picked up her diary and wrote: Thank you Father in Heaven for this day, even though it was horrible.

November 6th 2024

Wednesday was even worse than Tuesday. It turned out that the trip to the hospital had been in vain. Carlota was much worse, vomiting more and more.

In her huge room, lying on her bed, Carlota was writhing in more and more pain, horrible pain, and only cried softly.

Every now and then she would say: "Daddy, take me to your side. Please, ." Carlota loved her father, who had died in March of the previous year, and she couldn't forget her adored father. His death was traumatic for Carlota. That's why she had a photo of her father in her purse, another in her bedroom and another on the desk in her home office. She prayed to him every day and spoke to him often even though she knew he was dead.

Carlota's father had been an excellent father, husband, friend, with a beautiful life in the navy, without knowing what debt was, and with an absolutely fabulous life, so he left happily.

I always used to say to Carlota: "Daughter, if you need money, just say so..." Don't borrow money because the interest will eat at our table".

In that room and after a lot of vomiting, Helena turns to Carlota and says: "Carlota, don't you have the right to a doctor at home from the ACP?

Carlota replied:- Yes, I do.

-Then why don't you call?

She got up with great difficulty, clutching her cane, and went to her office. She turned on her computer, went to the Automóvel Clube de Portugal website and asked for a home doctor.

The service was excellent as always. And at four o'clock in the afternoon, Carlota, who had already fallen four times, but without actually fainting, received the doctor at her home from Porto.

Carlota was amazed at how quickly the doctor left Porto for Maceira da Lixa.

He was a tall man, with a stern, aloof air, but he looked very professional.

He looked at Carlota and saw that she was glassy-eyed, her eyes dark and sunken, like a living dead person.

He listened to her, took her blood pressure and then said: - You have severe dehydration, you're hypotensive and you need to go to hospital now. Carlota's blood pressure was 5 and her blood pressure was 7. Jesus!

He also said: - Today the INEM is more than 90 minutes late, so I want you to call the fire department here in the area and as soon as possible.

In fact, Carlota had seen on the news that on November 6, the INEM service was in absolute chaos and people had even died, and that the Minister of Health was going to order an inquiry.

Carlota called her goddaughter's husband, who had been her employee for more than ten years and lived nearby, then spoke to the doctor himself and received the necessary instructions from him and then called the Lixa Fire Brigade. He also said: "You can't go sitting in the ambulance, you have to lie on a stretcher."

Carlota thought: - What is this??! I'm really ill...... The doctor left a letter

for the hospital.

His letterhead read: Professor Doctor Tiago de Sousa Veloso, and then all his specialties.

Helena took the doctor's cell phone number.

Carlota thanked him for his very professional diagnosis and asked how much it was, to which he replied that the ACP would take care of it, and that he just wanted Carlota to get well.

A few minutes later he left.

In the meantime, Carlota fell again with a thud in the wide hallway of her house and could no longer get up. When the firemen arrived, they found her on the floor and helped her up, but with great difficulty. They then carried her slowly down the stairs of her house to the floor. A fall at that moment could have been fatal for Carlota.

They put Carlota on a stretcher and headed for Amarante hospital, her sister Helena also accompanying them in the ambulance.

Their blood pressure was really bad, dangerous, and they kept trying to get it to stabilize a bit with their own machine, which it eventually did.

 What's more, Carlota knew, because after graduating in Law, she had taken the Higher Course in Forensic Medicine, and she knew a little about some things in medicine, that low blood pressure more dangerous than high blood pressure and more difficult to restore to normal.

When they arrived at the Amarante Hospital emergency room, and after all the formalities, Carlota was given an orange bracelet and taken to an emergency room.

Carlota was terrified of needles, and suddenly she found herself being pricked everywhere, on both arms...for God's sake...what was that?

She was very nervous, next to her an old woman was moaning and screaming, Carlota's sister was sitting in a chair at the foot of her bed. She was distressed, it showed.

Carlota calmed down a little. And then she thought to herself: - Another half hour and I'd be dead. Dead at home.

The old lady looked at Carlota and said: - You suffer from anxiety. Calm down, breathe slowly, as if were blowing out a candle. And so Carlota did. She became calmer.

Carlota thought: - Blessed ACP. Blessed Doctor Tiago Veloso.

Blessedly, I pay a monthly fee of €9.30 to be a gold member of the ACP, which is what they call us, because there are various types of members with cheaper fees.

Blessedly, I paid 14 euros for the doctor to come to my house. No . Doctor Tiago Sousa Veloso had just saved her life.

She kept thinking to : "For God's sake, what is this? What has happened to me? I'm all pricked up, I've got a catheter and serum going through my veins!!!

A few minutes later, a doctor in her forties comes in, very friendly and turns to Carlota and says: - "You're seriously ill. How did you let it get to this point?"

Minutes later, Carlota went for a contrast CT scan of the brain. An hour and a half later, she went again for another contrast CT scan, but this time of the thorax.

His brain was a bit swollen and so was his heart. His diabetes was five hundred and something!

Well, after almost thirty years of not going to the doctor, because always felt fine, Carlota was now doing all the tests in one go, and a few more that she hadn't done in thirty years!

The doctor was afraid that Carlota had something wrong with her heart, so she decided to transfer her to Penafiel Hospital, which had all the specialties. There was no cardiology service in Amarante.

Carlota panicked. - What? I'm going to Penafiel.

I had seen several times on television and elsewhere that the news about Penafiel Hospital was not encouraging. Really bad news, with queues of people in the corridors of the emergency room, people hospitalized and catching bacteria, some of whom died.....

He turned to his sister and said: -Helena, they're taking me to Penafiel!

- What?

Carlota's sister panicked, she knew that Penafiel was not an easy hospital, it was a hospital that covered a very large population between Tâmega and Sousa and had a lot of patients.

She resigned herself and went home. The two sisters said goodbye through tears.

An hour later, with all the tests and clinical analyses already done, the doctor drew up a report for Penafiel and went in the ambulance to accompany Carlota along with a nurse . Wow! Carlota should to be monitored by the doctor who attended her in the emergency room.

On the way, the two of them talked, covering a distance of 26 km and taking about thirty-five minutes.

The doctor asked Carlota again how she had let herself go so far. That she was very ill.

They also talked about the courts and the case the doctor had against herself because of a patient who had died at her hands.

Carlota ended up calming the doctor down and giving her some good tips.

Penafiel Hospital - 23.30 hours

Emergencies

The ambulance carrying Carlota had just arrived. The doctor spoke to the head of the emergency department, who immediately said: - "We have no room. She has to stay outside in the corridor."

But in the meantime, after opening and reading the letter given to her by the doctor from Amarante who was accompanying Carlota, she sent Carlota's stretcher into the emergency room.

Carlota didn't even have time to say goodbye to that loving and attentive doctor.

 But she thought: -One day I'll visit you and thank you. And the nurse too, who was friendly, competent and whom Carlota had heard had worked in Barcelona.

Even though she was ill, Carlota was attentive to everything, to all the conversations, even those that took place quietly, attentive to all the noises and movements, so she heard everything the doctors and nurses said to each other.

Carlota had an eidetic memory and never forgot a face or feature.

The emergency room was in full swing that night of November 6th, with around thirty beds full of patients, in a large, huge room and then with a central station with computers and monitors were always beeping, and lots of nurses and doctors around them.

Carlota was in a bed, flanked by two other beds, one on each side with two elderly people.

I'd been stung again and , always having tests and analyses.

A doctor told her that it would take at least three hours to get the results.

Carlota felt exhausted and thirsty.

 She asked for water several times, but no one gave it to her because she was having more tests. She became increasingly thirsty and her mouth was dry.

She tried to sleep, but to no avail.

On his right side, the elderly man lying on the bed began: - Oh! Maria...Oh! Maria...Oh !Maria...constantly and without stopping.

Carlota could no longer hear the man. Then she shouted: -Shut up...shut up ...please shut up.

A nurse came up to the old man and said: - Be quiet, let the other patients sleep. He shut up, but only for a short time.

November 7th, 2024

It was Thursday morning. Carlota hadn't slept a wink. She asked for water again and nothing.

Half an hour later, he asked: ", please, give me water, please.

A nurse came in and said : - No , I can only wet her lips, and so she did.

But Carlota was still thirsty. How could they do this to her when they already knew that she had developed diabetes and that her thirst and dry mouth were a consequence?

Half an hour later, a cardiologist came to examine Carlota's heart.

An hour later he returned to make another.

And half an hour later, a saintly nurse gave Carlota a plastic cup full of water.

-WOW! Carlota felt like she was in paradise after drinking that glass water - For God's sake... thank you Lord.

Carlota was exhausted and restless. Suddenly a nurse approached Carlota, almost brought her face to face and said loudly: "Do want to die or do you want to be treated?

Jesus! What was that?

Carlota was carrying only her cell phone, her ID card and her St. Benedict's medal on her chest and asked to be allowed to them.

He didn't have a photo of his Father-in-Law with him. Nothing at all. Not even her book of daily prayers that always accompanied her.

Throughout the afternoon he had more heart tests.

He took two more bottles of saline. She was never given to eat. But Carlota wasn't hungry either, she was just extremely thirsty.

She was going to spend another night there, her second, and Carlota feared that it would be the same or worse than the previous one.

The old man continued that evening: - Oh Maria...Oh Maria...Oh Maria...

But this time Carlota didn't say anything, she didn't open her mouth, she let herself stay in that little cocoon that was her stretcher. And so she managed to get some sleep.

In the middle of the night, the emergency department received a new patient, a young man in his early twenties, shouting and uttering loud nonsense, like "ca....o", "f......e".

Christ. Carlota thought to herself. The peace was over.

Chapter 4

November 8th, 2024

Friday-10 a.m.

Carlota wakes up to the news from her cardiologist that her heart is fine. But she is accompanied by a doctor who tells her that she has DM - Diabetes Mellitus.

-"What?" asked Carlota.

-That's right. Do you have diabetes?

-Not that I know of.

-Does anyone have diabetes in their family?

-Not that I know of.

-Do you have any children?

-"No," replied Carlota dryly.

-But why? Because you couldn't or because you didn't want to?

-OH!!! Carlota , Carlota, was freaking out......

Carlota answered simply: - Because I didn't feel like it.

-Well, you have diabetes, here's some medicine for you to take.

-But Doctor, do you know if I have else? -asked Carlota fearfully.

The doctor was , he seemed to be saying .

And he replied dryly: - I don't know, I'm an endocrinologist and they called me just to tell you this.

She left with the cardiologist, who showed up an hour later to discharge Carlota.

Just like that. No more. Just like that.

Carlota left the hospital at noon, without a piece of paper, without a letter, without anything, without copies of all her tests. .

She called her sister to pick her up.

Half an hour later, Carlota was driving home in the car of her godson, who had come to pick her up.

He still looked as bad as before. He couldn't move.

When she got home, her godson Gonçalo helped her up the stairs and then Carlota went to bed. She was devastated.

Gonçalo was very frightened to see his godmother like this. A woman who had always been feisty, full of life, looked like a corpse.

He arrived at his parents' house distressed and said: - Mom, Dad, Caminda (the name she's called Carlota since she was a little girl, and that's how it's stayed) is so sick, so sick, you have to go and see her today without fail.

Carlota's goddaughter and her husband were distressed and went straight there.

 When they reached Carlota's room and saw her prostrate and white as lime, they were alarmed. They had never seen her like this.

Grace saw her godmother like that and said to her mother, Carlota's sister: Oh! Mom, Carlota's really ill, she's hit her hard, she's really hit her hard.....

Four days passed and Carlota was getting worse and worse, she kept vomiting non-stop.

Helena didn't know what else to say or do.

Then she thought of calling the ACP doctor, but he didn't answer.

November 12 and 13, 2024

Helena sent him a message, to which the doctor replied around midnight. The next day he arranged for Carlota to undergo a series of tests that he would prescribe and asked for them to be urgent.

Carlota received the prescription on her cell phone; she had never seen so many tests to do in her entire life.

Helena called a cab and went to Felgueiras Hospital. At the hospital they were amazed; they had never seen so many strange and weird tests carried out.

She asked for urgency and if they could go home.

The lady at the counter said yes, but she had to take the nurse home and bring her back. The nurse's service was free. They just had to take her and bring her back.

Helena paid for the tests, around €77.70! WOW... how expensive, but anyway.

He put the nurse in the cab, took her home, she took several vials of blood from Carlota and then took the cab back to the hospital.

The next day Carlota took a cab to pick them up from the emergency room, and paid 20 euros for an emergency appointment she didn't get!!!

The ACP doctor had asked to open it and see. The emergency doctor just said that the value was too high and it was wrong, it had to be around 7 and Carlota was 12!!!

What was that value? It was the so-called Glycated Hemoglobin (HbA1C) value, which was over 6.5%. It was serious.

Carlota arrived home and texted the results to the doctor.

On Wednesday the 13th, at around eighteen o'clock, Doctor Tiago Veloso called Carlota and told her that the problem was serious and that she had diabetic ketoacidosis and that she had to go to hospital now because only there could they treat her. They have to restore all the levels in Carlota's body to normal.

Carlota was startled and replied: -Doctor, I can't move now, can I go to the hospital tomorrow?

-If you don't want to go now, then go tomorrow.

Carlota went online to see what diabetic ketoacidosis was and was startled by what she read.

The person could fall into a coma and even die. WHAT?

For Good sake, what?

Carlota waited another hour, but then her sister came her room and said: - Carlota, we're not going to wait any longer, we're going to Penafiel Hospital now.

It was already eleven at night.

They called a cab and off they went, Carlota deciding that it would be quicker than calling the INEM. And so it was.

Carlota was devastated, grabbed her cane and got into the cab with her sister. She was in the front seat.

She was doing so badly, so badly, that the cab driver, who was already known to both of them and was always ready when needed, said: - Never in my life have I seen a doctor of that profession in such bad shape!

Carlota simply replied that being a doctor had nothing to do with her state of health.

The doctor had just saved Carlota again with his advice and wisdom.

When they arrived, they went straight to the emergency room, and after triage, they put an orange bracelet on Carlota and moved her from the wheelchair to a stretcher.

The nurse said that Carlota was reallybadly, very badly. Carlota replied that she had seen on the Internet that she could die.

Immediately, the nurse replied: - "Well, you all have the habit of going online to see what you're not supposed to."

Carlota was furious and replied at her wit's end: -Madam Nurse, I don't just watch anything on the Net, I know very well what I want to see and filter out what interests me.

The conversation ended right there.

Before going into the living room, Carlota was crying and only asked her sister not to lose her walking stick, so that she could keep it when she got home.

-Please Helena, please don't lose my cane.

-Rest assured, Carlota, I've already put her in the cab.

What was that cane that Carlota was so fond of?

It was Carlota's graduation cane. Her red cane from her graduation procession from the Faculty of Law of the University of Coimbra. WOW. Holy shit! That's right. A cane more than 33 years old! No wonder.

And why was that cane now appearing?

Because Carlota needed one to get around the house and she didn't have one. Would she really need to buy a normal cane?" she asked herself.

In fact, Carlota has many walking sticks from her walks and visits to Santigo de Compostela, where she also studied, after Coimbra, with her name engraved on some of them, but they aren't practical to help her walk more efficiently.

The graduation cane is made of strong wood and has a large curved handle. It was ideal for the moment.

And so much so that as soon as she was able to speak in the hospital, the first thing Carlota asked her sister was if the cane was in storage.

-"Of course," replied Helena.

Some nurses came to collect Carlota and took her to the same room where Carlota had been the first time.

 Only now she was further away and in a corner with a wall.

They connected her to a machine with a monitor and suddenly it beeping. Carlota sensed that she was falling apart, her oxygen was dropping rapidly, she could die at any moment.

Suddenly Carlota sees five distressed nurses her, poking here, poking there, one of them very sympathetically says: - "Excuse me, my dear, but it has to be done, this sting is going to hurt a lot, okay?"

But Carlota no longer wanted to know anything, she couldn't hear anything, it seemed to her that she was going to die right then and there.

He no longer cared what they did to his body, now he just wanted to die.

That Thursday morning was terrible, completely traumatizing.

Then there were more doctors, more tests, more stings, some of them successive, on the inside of my right wrist, on the edge of a small bone that we have there.

Those did hurt a lot and the doctors poked and prodded in search of the vein.

Oh my God...... how far you've come Carlota!!! Now you let them do everything to you. What an irony of fate.

Carlota was given serum, insulin and other liquids to restore all her values to normal, ions, protons and everything else.

An hour later, a very nice doctor administered insulin into her stomach and explained to Carlota that she had diabetes mellitus.

She already knew that Carlota was a specialist in international law, that she often traveled abroad (Carlota didn't know who had told the doctor this) mainly to Strasbourg, and that when she flew she couldn't take her insulin in the hold, but on her side.

He wished Carlota all the best, prescribed new medication and discharged her, as the previous pills made Carlota very sick and she refused them after three days.

Carlota was discharged around midday! She was only in hospital for twelve hours!

WOW!!! This time everything was so fast, efficient and with a fabulous medical team!!! Who would have done that?

Yes, this time Carlota could say with her mouth full, "Blessed is today's NHS!

Suddenly, at the back of the room, Carlota sees a group of people and a doctor asking questions and saying:- I want to know everything about Dr. Carlota.

Nurses and doctors who were in the group immediately asked: - Dr. Carlota? Who is Dr. Carlota?

They began to think and Carlota listened quietly in her corner, saying nothing.

 She was also petrified because the man next to her bed had just died of an epileptic seizure, right in front of her, without even a curtain separating the two beds.

How surreal! But it was the purest of truths. The man was shaking all over and no one even came to see him.

Carlota was so simple and so humble, even there in that hospital bed. Completely devoid of grandeur, of manias, and yet so important she was and is.

Suddenly a nurse stands up and says: - There's that lady at the back called Carlota Cardoso.

-       So it's really her - says the emergency director. - I want to know everything now. And she won't be discharged until everything has been sorted out so it doesn't happen like the first time!

-       How nice, Carlota thought to herself. Now she wondered why they hadn't treated her like this the first time. She still thinks about it today.

-

November 14th, 2024

Noon - Penafiel Hospital

Carlota left the hospital after meeting the diabetes nurse.

 She taught Carlota how to prick her insulin pen, how to prick her fingers and how to measure her capillary blood glucose every day and what the normal values are, and to be very strict in those procedures.

Carlota already here again, looking much better and clutching her beloved cane once more.

What a horrible two weeks it had been.

He arrived home and immediately put his cane down in his study, next to his red top hat, which he has kept with love and affection for thirty-three years, as it was signed inside on the day of the procession by many illustrious figures, some of them his teachers.

 Carlota's hat bore the signatures of the late Lucas Pires, Perez de Cuellar, who at the time was the Secretary General of the UN and had come to Coimbra to visit the Faculty of Law, and the signature of MárioSoares, Orlando de Carvalho, the fearsome professor of Real Rights, Figueiredo Dias, the professor of Criminal Law and the Rector, Professor Rui Alarcão, who signed Carlota's Diploma, among others.

And Carlota's top hat was very special indeed, because on the night of the 5th grade parade, the car her class, with the wind and speed, the top hat off Carlota's head.

-OHH!!! For God's sake, what now?

Carlota's hat had flown into a large, very tall tree inside a boarding house on the avenue by the River Mondego.

They all got out of the car and went straight to the owner of the boarding house, who, seeing Carlota crying copiously, let them go to the tree to get the hat, but it was too high.

What should we do now? One of Carlota's colleagues thought of the Coimbra Fire Brigade

. - That's right," they all said in unison.

They went to the fire station, which granted Carlota's request.

And minutes later, they were all hanging from the fire engine, their suits and top hats flying.

Half an hour passed, and then the firemen brought Carlota's hat down with a crane.

Carlota was overjoyed. She would be grateful for life. And so much so that the next day the Diário de Coimbra newspaper carried a front-page photograph of the fire engine with Carlota hanging from the car with her top hat on her head and her friends next to her.

And the newspaper headline simply said:

"Soldiers of PEACE from Coimbra save a law student's top hat".

 Carlota religiously keeps a copy of this newspaper.

WOW! Carlota, you have so many good things in life, so many fabulous, unique memories. Why do you want to die? Damn.

After putting down his cane, he went to his desk and picked up his diary. He hadn't written in it since November 4th. Oh my God!

In the meantime, she picks up the phone and receives the terrible news that Dona Beatriz de Vasconcelos, aged 93, has died.

 She was one of Carlota's biggest clients and friends, as were her daughters, especially her daughter Manuela de Lemos Vasconcelos, a big businesswoman in the textile sector for whom Carlota worked.

She felt sad and cried. She had died the day before, on the 13th, and Carlota was in hospital. He couldn't say goodbye to her or go to the funeral, and he realized that he wouldn't even be able to attend the seventh-day mass.

God, how bad, how sad Carlota was.

 When she got well, the first thing she would do would be to visit Dona Beatriz, who now lived in a private family chapel next to her husband in the Lanhoso cemetery.

 Beatriz was a very wealthy lady, but she was extremely simple and great. She adored Carlota and even said that she was her third daughter.

Carlota also adored Dona Beatriz de Vasconcelos and would miss her terribly.

He opened his diary to November 4th and wrote: very ill. Day 5 very ill. Day 6, day 7 very ill in hospital and so he wrote down all the missing days until November 14.

Every day she wrote at the end: "Thank you Jesus for these days, as horrible as they were.

Then he checked that he hadn't spent any money in all those days. Jesus: zero euros spent. Not even a coffee in the street.

Really, if you don't leave the house, you spend zero. Zero.

Then he wrote: cab fares, 200 euros, pharmacy and doctors, more than 600 euros.

A month without work and Carlota had to go to her savings. She had to start working again quickly.

At the bottom of the diary page on that November 14th, Carlota wrote in fuzzy letters:

BEGINNING OF A NEW LIFE

Ironically, do readers of this book know what day November 14th is? WORLD DIABETES DAY.

Carlota spent the most horrible ten days of her life. But she came out of it alive, unscathed and with a terrible chronic illness for the rest of her life. She would have to live with it. Would she succeed?

Only time would tell.

Chapter 5

Carlota's new life

November 15th, 2024

Carlota went out on the street for the first time, she wanted to drive, to see how she was doing she took her beloved cane to help her walk down the street.

She went with her sister to the center of Lixa to do some new shopping now that Carlota had to eat very different things. She bought low-fat, sugar-free yogurts, sugar-free cookies, low-fat milk, which she already drank, wholemeal pasta and zero-calorie cola.

WOW! No cakes, no juice, no coffee, no sugar. But lots of vegetables, oh yes lots of vegetables.

Half an hour later, she felt very tired and drove home very slowly.

Not bad for a start.

Professor Guilhermina Rego called the next day as soon as she heard that Carlota was out of hospital. After a long conversation, she said to Carlota: -"Dr. Carlota has chronic diabetes. There's no cure for that. What have you been doing? Now you have to be very careful, very rigorous, just the rigor you apply every day in your profession and in law. All of us who know you need you very much, Doctor, you are very much missed."

Carlota thanked her for the call and was very touched. But the truth is that Doctor. Guilhermina's words never left mind.

He remembers them every day.

However, the days went by and they weren't easy.

Carlota fell into a state of depression, catching up with her sister almost every day, because of the pills, because she was drinking too little water, because she was letting herself go downhill.

And because of the pills that made her nauseous, Helena started sneaking them to Carlota, crushed in her breakfast bread or in her milk, and she didn't notice.

But a week later, with pain in her conscience, Helena confessed to Carlota what she had been doing. But she said nothing, didn't reproach her or get angry. From that day on, Carlota started taking them and got used to them.

And getting into it bravely with Helena was the worst thing they could do to Carlota, who was simply devastated. Helena was everything to Carlota, her safe haven, and they rarely got angry with each other.

Carlota went to Google to look up things about diabetes, but she didn't know how to speak.

 She couldn't see any sites, because the web was full of unreliable sites. Information about diabetes abounded on the web like wild mushrooms growing in the forests.

A lot of the news was devastating: you could die, you could fall into a coma, you could have your lower limbs amputated, you could go blind, you could get diabetic feet.........Jesus!!!

Carlota was even more horrified. And more afraid. And she went back to her previous paranoia: she would rather die.

She turned to her sister in tears and said: - I'm finished Helena, I'm finished.

- My life is over, it has no meaning. What am I doing here?

Helena, furious and desperate to see Carlota like this, replied harshly: - "If you want to die, kill yourself at once.

Helena did this so that her sister would react and not let herself apart.

Another week passed, with ups and downs, and on the 21st Carlota had a dinner with a very important client, where one of the lawyers she worked with would be present.

Dinner had already been postponed twice and could not be postponed any longer.

It was urgent and Carlota had to go, and on top of that they had a trial for this company the following day, the 22nd, at ten o'clock in Felgueiras. It was a continuation and Carlota had to go too.

I was nervous about those days.

Carlota was doing everything right and with absolute rigor, taking her insulin in the morning, then breakfast, then the pill and then lots of finger pricks during the day.

Carlota was becoming addicted to the bites, sometimes doing eight a day and spending a lot of money on ribbons and picks.

-Jesus, Carlota! Stop a . His sister and some friends said.

But it felt like an addition, the fact that I always wanted to check my blood glucose levels.

And if they were high, then Carlota became very distressed and very nervous.

And the rigor that Carlota implemented in her life made her give up sugar for good on November 14th.

 When she was in the office in Felgueiras, she would sometimes go to the café for breakfast, but she gave that up for good.

She stopped drinking coffee, which she loved, but was afraid of, at least until she went to her family doctor's appointment.

She gave up all kinds of cakes and the white bread she loved. She only ate dark bread and rye bread, no cereal or wholemeal bread.

WOW!!! What is this Carlota?

Everyone in the family was completely stunned by such a radical change. They wondered if it would always be like this or if after a few months Carlota would regress and go back to sweets.

But after what she saw every day, Sister Helena was absolutely certain that Carlota would not turn back. And she told her daughter and son-in-law.

In the pivotal week when she had to go to dinner and the trial the next day, Carlota dared to walk without a cane and to go out alone without it and without her sister's company.

She realized that she still had to go down and up the stairs, one by one, because one thing she soon realized was that her legs hurt a lot, they burned and itched. They were strange, horrible pains.

She spoke to a doctor friend who told her it was normal at first.

Even so, Carlota was sad, and she was even sadder when she had to climb onto a low stool to get to the top cupboard in the kitchen.

Carlota put her right foot on the bench and then tried to climb onto the bench with her second, but she couldn't bend her left leg to do so.

-Ups! What is this? She was even more frightened and thought: my legs be paralyzed? She was terrified again. In fact, every day was a surprise, with good things and bad.

But this week was crucial for Carlota and on Thursday she got all dressed up to go to dinner. She met the client at the factory, left her car in the company car park and drove off in the client's car.

The client was a 73-year-old man, a big shoe entrepreneur, who drove a Mercedes S-Class, the latest model and fabulous. Carlota loved cars.

The journey went smoothly, the client drove safely and efficiently and it seemed as if Carlota was in a cradle.

He even remarked to his sister afterwards that of all the trips he had made with clients driving, that trip and drive had been the best of all in his life.

During the trip the client asked Carlota if she was feeling better, he had been very worried about her, which Carlota thanked him for, and then she felt she could open up completely and decided to tell him that she had developed diabetes and was very sad.

The client immediately replied:- "Doctor Carlota, don't look like that, I've had diabetes for twenty-something years. I was diagnosed at the age of 52 and I'm here fresh as a whistle.

- For many years I didn't go to the doctor because I was healthy, but then this happened. I take the pen in the morning with the insulin, 14 units, two tablets a day, one in the morning and one in the evening, and I have a device on my arm to measure my blood sugar.

Carlota became a little more animated. She explained what she was doing too, but she was taking 16 U and only one pill a day.

They had arranged to go from Felgueira to Porto to eat grilled fish, but then it didn't turn out as they had thought.

Even so, Carlota didn't eat any starters, while the others ate melon, ham and snacks. Lie: Carlota ate two codfish cakes, but didn't touch the wine, she always drank water, then she ate grilled sea bass with two potatoes, carrots and vegetables and for dessert she ate pineapple but then stopped because it didn't taste good.

He resisted not drinking coffee and not even decaf.

WOW! Carlota, you did very well," she said to herself.

She got home at midnight and was very tired. But I'm glad she did, because it was Carlota who knew the whole process well. Everything had gone perfectly.

The next day, Carlota got dressed up again to go to the Felgueiras trial of the same company. She got ready and took her new prop along with her purse and briefcase.

 And what was it?

A bag containing a thermos with hot water, a box of cookies,a clementine, your chopping board and the appropriate ribbons.which Carlota called straws, and two packets of sugar because her blood sugar was below 70.

Every day she took this bag with her when she went out, only changing the piece of fruit.

 And this was because Carlota had been told that she had to eat at least every two hours and, in fact, when two hours passed, Carlota's body would send her signals, she would start shaking a lot, she would feel like she was going to faint and she would only calm down when she put something in her mouth.

My God, Carlota, what a life you have now!

Halfway through the trial where he was advising the lawyer, he had to go out for a bite to eat and a drink, he was getting used to his new life.

Another stage has been reached.

Chapter 6

The days went by and the month of November, the most horrible November of his entire life, had no way of ending.

One day, Carlota forgot to take her pill and couldn't take it in the afternoon. She panicked and didn't tell her sister until much later, when she became angry and distressed.

To remedy the situation, Carlota decided to set a daily alarm on her smartphone to remind her to take her pill. Thanks God.

A few more days passed and Carlota went out with her sister and forgot to take her insulin, which is the first thing she does in the morning.

They went back after half an hour to take their insulin. My God, it was a lot to take in.

In the meantime, Carlota had read in a CUF study that nerves and stress were a major cause of diabetes. And Carlota was very anxious and schismatic, in addition to her intense working life.

In the first few days back, Carlota had poor eyesight, blurred vision, headaches and difficulty writing.

She got scared and even wondered if she had become less intelligent. It seemed that she couldn't think, but she was wrong, it was just tiredness and she wasn't completely cured yet.

A few days later, she commented on this to Professor Guilhermina, who, as soon as she heard Carlota's outburst, laughed and said that Carlota would never suffer from this ailment, of that she was sure. Carlota was happy with that answer and became much more cheerful.

On the penultimate day of November, Carlota wanted to go to Porto to see her mother, as they both missed each other terribly.

After coming from Madrid, Carlota received an invitation from an important lawyer in Felgueiras. After many trips from Port to Felgueiras and vice versa, she decided to move to Macieira da Lixa, as her house was only six kilometers from the lawyer's office, which also had an office in Porto.

But Carlota went on to manage the Felgueiras office. It was wonderful, she spent almost no money on gas, paid no tolls, paid no parking fees, always parked outside the office and didn't waste time in traffic jams.

WOW! Could there be a better paradise?

Then Carlota became very fond of Maceira da Lixa, she loved living there, in the daily quiet, in the immense quiet of the weekends, walking her dogs in the garden. The noise of the birds, the roosters crowing, the church bell telling the time.

It was wonderful to live in the Province, as silly as many people say it is.

Carlota didn't care about the fools, she didn't talk to the neighbors much either and was very reserved, just like her sister.

Then he had a huge office inside his house and he often stayed there to work, and he produced much more in that peace and quiet. when it came to writing, he felt like he was in paradise, and inspiration came flooding in.

Five years in Macieira da Lixa, Carlota began to stop thinking about her beloved city of Porto.

 She didn't miss anything, everything was cheaper, the food, fruit and vegetables from the farmers, which were truly organic and cheap!!!

And the meat was the same, straight from the pasture. The fish was more expensive, because it had to come from the coast.

Everything was harmony, peace and tranquillity.

However, Carlota's mother, already elderly, was a very independent lady and anyone who took away her house in Porto and lived in Porto would be like killing her.

He would often come to spend a few days in Macieira da Lixa, but then he would return to his little house in Porto, in Virtudes, the historic area of Porto, close to the Palace of Justice.

And as long as her mother remained healthy and independent, Carlota would never commit the atrocity of taking her mother away from the city of Porto and her home. She was sure that if she did, her mother wouldn't last long and Carlota would never forgive herself if she did.

Chapter 7

Carlota went with her sister to see their mother. She left at around 9.30 in the morning, so as not to hit any heavy traffic at the tollbooths.

 The journey was quick, but after the toll, and on the VCI, Carlota took another forty minutes, and then from the Palácio de Cristal to Virtudes it took another half hour.

That was enough to make Carlota nervous, and when she got to her mother's house, she had a bite and was 209 with diabetes!!! And she had left home with 124!!!

She got scared. She had to find a way to control her nerves.

She hugged her mother with great longing and they both cried. An hour later, Carlota left with her sister and her mother and went for lunch near their home, on Passeio das Virtudes.

 The three of them ate a steak on bread which was fabulous, with no sauces, and each drank a natural cola zero. They didn't have coffee.

Then Carlota and her sister returned home. It was about fifteen o'clock in the afternoon, and to get out of Oporto.

Carlota found herself stuck again, the exit to Ermesinde and the tollbooth was in full swing.

It was enough to get on his nerves again and when he got home his blood sugar was over 250, he was 274!!! And over 250 was serious.

She then called the diabetes nurse at Penafiel Hospital. She calmed Carlota down and said that it was normal, but if the levels

if they remained high for more than eight days, then I would have to go to hospital.

However, the next day everything was back to normal and Carlota was more cheerful.

The beginning of December started with Carlota working almost 100%. Her eyesight had improved, her reasoning and thinking were as good as , at their best, but she was still a little tired. But it wasn't for nothing, Carlota still hadn't recovered for a month.

The morning sickness disappeared, largely because Carlota was taking, on the advice of a vascular surgeon known to her sister, a gastric protector called "PARIET", which was truly miraculous.

It was the first medicine Carlota took early in the morning and on an empty stomach.

Carlota was now feeling more energized, she was back to working hard, more new cases were coming up, but now she was trying not to get so worked up.

It was an arduous task, but I was succeeding. WOW!

The friends were amazed but happy.

So were the clients. When Carlota went out to lunch with clients, out of respect they would refuse to order desserts, but Carlota always said that it didn't affect her, that they could eat as much as they liked.

Carlota resisted starters, wines and sweets, and even very sweet fruit.

She loved mango but now knew she had to avoid it at all costs because it was too sweet. She gave it up for good.

When she went to buy bread, Carlota resisted those shop windows full of sweets, cakes and everything else.

I honestly didn't feel like eating anything.

Now that Christmas was upon us, Carlota was aware of what was coming, but she knew she had the strength to resist all kinds of sweets and she was sure she could do it.

Chapter 8

Carlota thus went through atrocious, indescribable suffering that she would not wish on anyone.

I still wasn't afraid of dying, but what I didn't want, and what was quite different, was the fact that I would never again go through what I had gone through in those ten days.

Carlota stopped drinking the water from the rocks, which she used to drink a lot, but with this illness she was now terrified of vomiting. Just the thought of vomiting terrified her.

 She remembered the pain in her digestive system caused by vomiting.

By God, that's what you didn't want in your life. Never again.

Then he realized that his palate had changed.

 He used to love cold drinks, but many still had to have ice in them and now he couldn't drink cold or iced drinks. All he liked now was hot water, not warm but hot.

He ate lunch and drank hot water, snacked and drank hot water, and always had a thermos with tea or hot water and unsweetened cookies on his desk.

When I went out, the same bottle always carried hot water or hot tea.

What is this, Carlota? - he asked .

Carlota couldn't explain, she didn't have an answer to that question. All she knew was that she now loved hot water and that it tasted like life.

Then she couldn't eat pineapple or pineapple, which was another fruit she loved. But now, as well as tasting bad, it gave him heartburn.

My God, Carlota, you really have to prepare yourself for a new life that's very different from the one you had before," -she thought to herself.

One day at home, Carlota and her sister decided to do a radical clean-out of the kitchen cupboards and pantry.

First, he threw away everything that was already open and grafted and that he couldn't eat, even throwing a lot of it into the fields for the stray cats.

Goodbye jams, goodbye chocolates, goodbye Milka cookies, goodbye white pasta, goodbye packets of potato chips, goodbye burguers, goodbye ham, goodbye sausages, goodbye Iberian ham.......Oh!!! For God's sake, what am I going to eat now?

Then she decided to give everything she had left to the neighbors who lived next door and whom she loved very much.

The cupboards are empty and the fridge has almost all gone the same way.

Carlota was now saying goodbye to sausages, processed meats and red meat, among other things.

She started eating more turkey and rabbit, which were precisely two of the meats she hated the most. But she had to, if Carlota really wanted to achieve the rigor she had set herself and promised herself.

And with this rigor came new habits, such as always eating Jell-O for dessert, something I used to hate. And I used to buy Jell-O with zero sugar.

Rigor at breakfast, always with milk and granulated coffee with cereal and toasted rye bread with unsalted butter.

 That's how it was every day, and that's how it would be.

Then I always tried to eat at the same times of day to establish a routine. Eating at the right time was essential for a diabetic.

He ate every two and a half hours, so he ate at least six meals a day, and tried to sleep soundly at night, not going more than eight hours a night without eating.

I had read that sleep was essential and that lack of sleep a sign of diabetes, as were insomnia and severe tremors.

Carlota realized that over the last few months she'd been sleeping very little, she'd spent hours at a time at night without sleeping, all the time, walking around the house without getting any sleep.

And Carlota was rigorous, whether she was at home all day, out on the road working or even out for a walk.

If she was and about, she'd go to the usual restaurant, which was not only cheap during the week, but always made healthy food for Carlota. It was the restaurant she frequented even with her work colleagues and where most of the shoe entrepreneurs went, many of whom Carlota worked for.

If I was at home, I'd start cooking around noon minus a quarter so that I'd be eating around 12:30.

Then, religiously, he would let two hours pass and go for a bite to check on his diabetes after lunch and record them in his little book.

 Around 3.30 in the afternoon I'd have a bite to eat, then around five another bite, then another half an hour and a snack, and so on. I'd have dinner at nine in the evening and then read for a while and go to bed.

He always got up at least seven o'clock in the morning, took his first fasting bite, wrote it down in his little book, took his insulin before breakfast and then the terrible pill.

This was Carlota's routine until she felt that her diabetes would totally under control.

She knew that diabetes couldn't be cured, but it could be reduced a lot and controlled in such a way that in the future, maybe even Carlota could stop taking insulin and just take pills.

And Carlota got it into her head that she was going to do everything she could to make that happen, so that she would at least stop taking insulin. There was a long way to go.

Chapter 9

Carlota, who hadn't been to the family doctor until then, wrote a letter to her doctor, who was the doctor for the whole family, asking her to see her, and enclosed all the documentation she had, tests, discharge from hospital and the medication she was taking.

Two days later, Carlota received a message saying that she had a nursing appointment and a general medicine appointment at 8.30 in the morning.

WOW! Carlota, who until then hadn't wanted to go to the doctor, was now anxious and dying to go.

What an irony of fate! There really is a first time for everything.

On the day of her appointment, Carlota left home almost an hour early. Then, inside the health center, she couldn't for her turn to come.

When it was her turn, she first went to the nurse's appointment, where the nurse explained everything to her: how to care for her feet, cut her toenails, make sure her shoes were free of stones, etc.

Then he had to measure his blood pressure twice a week and write it down on a chart he was given.

A few minutes later, he went to see his doctor.

 It was the perfect appointment. Right from the start there was an empathy between the two. Carlota was impressed by her wisdom, experience and professionalism.

The same happened with the doctor's vision of Carlota, who was a person with a lot of knowledge, a lot of culture and very realistic.

He immediately understood Carlota's attitude and how she must have felt when she was diagnosed with diabetes.

-"You know, Doctor Carlota, I often say that ignorance is a blessing, because when you have little or no knowledge, it's easier to accept the disease."

-"Now for a person like you, it's awful, never having been ill and now having this on top of you."

-"Believe me, if you were told that you had cancer, everyone would understand and feel sorry for you...."

-"Now say, you have diabetes, everyone says, oh! lots of people have diabetes, it's nothing special and so on...".

-"But it's not like that, diabetes is dangerous and terrible and it's not easy to live with it, and even less so in the early stages that you're in."

Carlota was stunned by that explanation and by the doctor's understanding. That was exactly the reasoning.

Everyone told Carlota that it wasn't so bad, but it was just talk and nothing more.

And when Carlota took the course she did, many people said that when they appear, everyone reacts like that because we're all afraid of dying.

But Carlota didn't think so and told the doctor so.

Carlota continued say that she wasn't afraid of dying, but she was afraid of suffering and never wanted to go through the atrocious suffering she had experienced again.

And it was this horrible suffering that made Carlota rethink her life, establish new priorities, think differently, and if she already led a frugal life, now she would be even more so.

His motto was to live one day at a time and now it will be more like that, one day at a time and we'll see.

The ten terrible days she spent there were a real lesson for Carlota.

Ten days that completely turned Carlota's whole life upside down.

Later, lying in her bed, she thought about what would have happened if she had died.

By God, he hadn't even made a will, and he did it so often for his clients, so that they would be protected by his assets.

Carlota didn't, she had nothing protected, and her other spiteful sister was going to take everything that was hers, apart from the things that belonged to her sister Helena, which Carlota had won by hand.

- My God

!!! -she said to . Not that.

He was going to make his will as soon as possible, even if he lived to be a hundred.

Those ten days were a life lesson for Carlota, a very hard lesson and Carlota had already had many bad and bitter moments in her life, very tough situations that she had always overcome with hard work, resilience and a lot of faith, but none like those ten days.

I was going to do everything I could to make sure it never happened .

END

Tips and advice for people with diabetes

There's a lot to read and see on the web, but it's not always the most accurate or correct.

We'll always have to filter the news and information, and we'll always have a family doctor to accompany us.

We can always consult a specialist, an endocrinologist, to give us support for our health, but the family doctor will always be the main advisor, the one who gives us medication and prescriptions, the one who regulates and stabilizes the values in ml, the doses we should take of insulin, or raise or lower those doses.

Just as it will always be the family doctor who will tell us which pills are best to take, and from time to time we should have our blood tested to check our blood glucose levels, this is the value that needs to be strictly controlled so that we don't have a situation that gets complicated tomorrow.

People with diabetes should eat a healthy diet.

Meals for diabetics should always be a pleasurable time, even if we are prevented from eating certain things.

But food made well, with love and pleasure, with little salt, no fat and no sauces, will always be a pleasant moment.

You just have to want it.

Nowadays, there are so many foods that are good for diabetics, even without salt, little salt or sugar, which is our worst enemy.

We just have to be very careful with foods that claim to be sugar-free but then have saccharin, which is even worse.

We should avoid sweeteners, which are terrible substitutes for sugar but make it worse and many of which contain carcinogenic substances.

We should avoid foods that have the word "light" written on them, because this is even worse than sugar.

Diabetics should avoid eating too many carbohydrates such as rice and white pasta. But they can be eaten from time to .

Many people prefer wholemeal pasta, but contrary to what people think, wholemeal pasta also contains sugar, but here the sugar goes

It is more slowly absorbed by the body, unlike white pasta.

You should eat plenty of vegetables as well as fruit, but those that contain less sugar.

Mangoes, grapes, figs, melons and bananas should be avoided because they are very sweet fruits.

Alcoholic drinks should be avoided, but you can have a good wine every now and then.

Beer, especially craft beer, is good and doesn't cause any danger. As for the terrible

sweets, they should be eradicated from our lives.

With the evolution of the disease and its sort of cure, cure in the sense of effective diabetes control, then yes, we can eat a good sweet from far and wide.

Other tips for living with diabetes

Diabetics should lead a calm life, and know how to control anxiety and stress.

They should exercise, if not in the gym, then by taking walks and going outdoors.

For those who like it, they can practice yoga, meditation, therapeutic writing or even, for those who have the ability, creative writing, reading books of various kinds, novels, historical romance, thrillers, comics, medical books, self-help books, among others.

Those who have faith must cultivate moments of introspection, of conversations with God, of talking to Jesus who always listens to us.

Going to a church, even if we're alone inside, so that we can meet God, you can be sure that we'll come out of there much better.

For those who profess other religions, seek your God, your faith, and you too will be heard and cared for.

For those who are agnostic, may they search within themselves for the reflection that they believe will open doors to the strength they need to overcome this illness and move on.

 We all have an inner Strength within us that will certainly help overcome all adversity.

As someone once said, a life without hardship and adversity is like distilled water, it has no taste.

Finally: Mr. Diabetes, let's do it, let's fight it with all due respect.

Macieira da Lixa

December 8th, 2024

www.ingramcontent.com/pod-product-compliance
Lightning Source LLC
Chambersburg PA
CBHW031435250726
48656CB00002B/995